THE PLANTAR FASCIITIS BOOK

Dr. Donald Pelto

Table of Contents

INTRODUCTION

Thank you for your interest in the "The Plantar Fasciitis Book" This book is intended to help provide further education to you about plantar fasciitis.

By no means do we believe that this book takes the place of visiting the office. However, it can be used as a good **reference source for information** about treatments that you can do at home and what treatments are used in the office setting.

To view about other learning resources about plantar fasciitis, go to www.drpelto.thinkific.com.

To your health,

Dr. Donald Pelto.

PLANTAR FASCIITIS

What is Plantar Fasciitis?

Plantar fasciitis is an inflammation of the muscle under the heel which can cause intense heel pain. This can also be called heel spur syndrome when a spur is present on an x-ray evaluation. Heel pain can also be due to other causes such as a stress fracture, tendonitis, arthritis, nerve irritation or even a bone cyst. Since there are many possible causes, it is essential to have the heel pain properly diagnosed.

Symptoms of Plantar Fasciitis

The most common symptoms of plantar fasciitis are:

- Pain on the bottom of the heel
- Pain first thing in the morning when getting out of bed
- Pain that increases over time

People with plantar fasciitis often describe the pain as severe upon rising in the morning and then improving as they become more active during the day. After they sit down and relax, their pain is lessened until they begin moving again. After walking for a few minutes, the pain decreases because they are stretching the plantar fascia. For other people the pain is worse when they are on their feet for long periods of time.

The Plantar Fasciitis Scorecard®

To help you better understand your symptoms, I have put together a Plantar Fasciitis Score Card. To use this scorecard read each of the items on the column on the left and rank your symptoms and give it a score. Add the scores you have on the right column and read the information below.

Plantar Fasciitis Scorecard®

		1	2	3	4	5	6	7	8	9	10	11	12	Score
1	Severity Of Symptoms	I don't have any pain with my plantar fascia at this time.			I have pain when I do extended periods of standing and walking but besides that I don't have daily pain.			I have pain daily when walking and standing.			I have pain all the time when standing and walking despite all treatments and it even hurts when sitting down now.			
2	Length Of Symptoms	I have had symptoms for a few days to a week but they have gone away.			I have had symptoms for a week to a month.			I have had symptoms for 1 to 6 months.			I have had symptoms between one to two years.			
3	Morning Pain	I don't have any pain when getting up in the morning.			I have occasional pain to my heel when getting up in the morning but it goes away after a few minutes.			I have pain every day when I get up in the morning or after sitting and driving but it goes away.			I have pain every day when I get up and the pain does not go away at all unless I am sitting down.			
4	Effects On Lifestyle	My plantar fasciitis does not affect my lifestyle I can do anything that I want. I am very active.			I only notice my heel pain when I and walking for longer periods or exercising but I can "push through."			I have pain daily but I can still work and do my daily activities.			All I can think about is pain. My work is affected because of constant pain and I stopped working out.			
5	Weight Gain and Activity Level	I have had no weight gain and no change in my activity level with plantar fasciitis.			I have gained a few pounds and am exercising less due to my heel pain.			I have gained 5-10 pounds and my activity level is greatly reduced but I am still able to work and walk around.			I can't do anything because of my heel pain and have gained over 20 pounds since my symptoms began.			
6	Understanding About Plantar Fasciitis	I am interested in learning about my condition and I regularly see my doctor for treatment			I have have a good grasp about what causes plantar fasciitis and am eager to learn more about the condition.			I have "Googled" my condition and talked to some people about plantar fasciitis.			I am not interested in learning about my condition and think my doctor should be able to do everything.			
7	Effects On Attitude	I have no problem and don't feel like my plantar fasciitis affects my attitude.			I have a few bad days because of my heel pain but I am hopeful the symptoms will get better with time.			I am aggravated at how long I am having my symptoms despite actively trying to get better.			I feel depressed because of how debilitating my plantar fasciitis is and I am not sure what to do to get better.			
8	Shoe Gear	I can go barefoot and wear any shoes that I want without any problems.			I feel better with shoes that are more supportive.			When I am barefoot I have pain but as long as I have shoes on I feel better and can be more active.			I have pain with shoes and without shoes. There is nothing that is comfortable for me.			
	Scorecard	⬇			⬇			⬇			⬇			

Scoring System

0-24 - You probably don't have a problem with plantar fasciitis at this time, but you may have had a problem in the past. You don't need any treatment but would benefit from wearing supportive shoes as well as foam rolling on your own.

25-48 - You have mild symptoms of plantar fasciitis. You may be able to treat this on your own with some of the home therapies or treatments recommended below. If the pain becomes worse or more bothersome, you should probably get help from a podiatrist.

49-72 - You have severe symptoms and are probably already getting treatment. If you are not receiving treatment, you would benefit from treatment to help resolve your symptoms more quickly. The information below will help you start your own treatment before seeking professional advice.

73-96 - You have very severe plantar fasciitis and need help urgently. You may have other conditions along with plantar fasciitis as well and should be seeking help from a professional. You may be a candidate for advanced treatments or surgery.

Causes of Plantar Fasciitis

The most common cause of plantar fasciitis is too much motion in your foot, causing excess pulling on the plantar fascia. The plantar fascia is a ligament-like structure that runs from the heel to the ball of your foot. When your foot has too much motion there is excess force pulling on the plantar fascia causing it to become inflamed. Feet that are overly flat (pronated) or have too much of an arch are more likely to develop plantar fasciitis.

Also, an overly tight Achilles tendon (equinus) in the back of your leg will cause excess tightness on the structures on the bottom of the foot. If you imagine two ropes pulling on the heel bone, the bottom one is the plantar fascia and the top one is the Achilles tendon. If the Achilles is pulling up, the plantar fascia will naturally become tighter making it more prone to injury.

Wearing non-supportive footwear on hard, flat surfaces puts an abnormal amount of strain on the plantar fascia and can also lead to plantar fasciitis. This is especially true for those that wear flip-flops over extended periods of time and for those who have a job that requires long hours on their feet. Obesity can also contribute to plantar fasciitis.

Diagnosis

To properly evaluate heel pain, a complete medical history and examination of the mechanics of your foot and lower extremity mechanics is necessary. This will require an evaluation of your walking (gait) and possible video or photography of your feet. By doing this we can rule out all other possible causes of plantar fasciitis.

Also, diagnostic imaging such as **x-ray, ultrasound, bone scan, and magnetic resonance imaging** (MRI) may be used to distinguish among different types of heel pain. Sometimes x-rays can reveal heel spurs with people with plantar fasciitis. However, these spurs are rarely a source of pain.

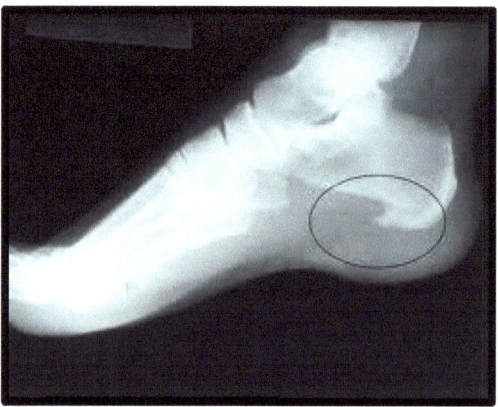

Figure 1: X-ray of heel spur

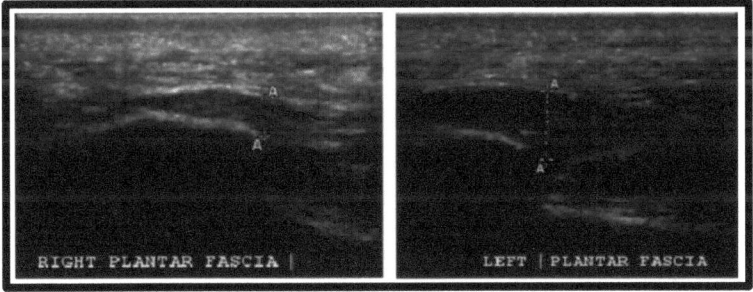

Figure 2: Ultrasound of plantar fascia showing thickness increased on the left side

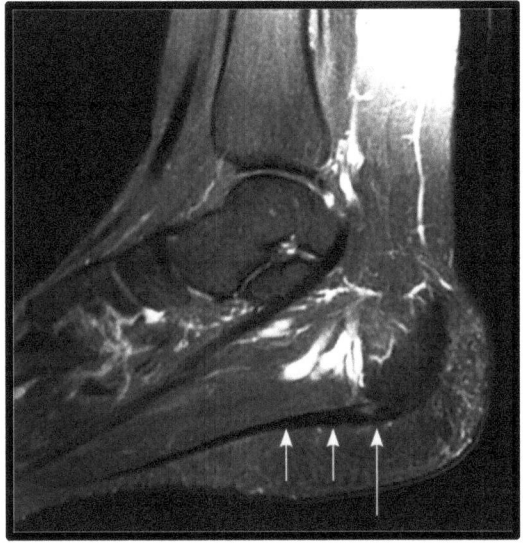

Figure 3: MRI of plantar fascia showing thickening and inflammation

Plantar Fasciitis Treatment Evaluator®

Here is the Plantar Fasciitis Treatment Evaluator® I put together that evaluates the different treatments based on their results (Reducing Inflammation, Reducing Tightness, Stabilizing Foot and Reducing Pressure) and effectiveness. This is essential because many people who read about different treatments think that all are similarly effective, which is incorrect.

Icing is not as effective as a cortisone injection yet both work at reducing inflammation. Similarly, supportive shoes are not as effective as custom orthotics in stabilizing your foot. However, when wading through the material presented either online or by your physician, it may be difficult determining what treatment to try first.

I hope you find the Plantar Fasciitis Treatment Evaluator® helpful in determining the best type of treatment for your plantar fascial pain. The following resources are in order of effectiveness based on the table below

Plantar Fasciitis Treatment Evaluator®

Effectiveness Scale (5 is most effective)	Reduce Inflammation	Reduce Tightness	Stabilize Foot and Reduce Pressure
5 – Most Effective	Cortisone Injection	Physical Therapy	Custom Orthotics
4	Shockwave Therapy		Walking Boot
4	Amniotic Membrane Therapy		
3 – Moderately Effective	Steroid Anti-Inflammatory Medications (Prednisone)	Home Therapy (Foam Rolling, Stick and TP Tools)	Over-the-Counter Arch Support
3	Oral Non-Steroidal Anti-Inflammatory Medications (Motrin, Ibuprofen)		Supportive Shoes
3			Strapping of Foot
2	Icing and Contrast Baths	Stretching	Padding
2	Platelet Rich Plasma	Night Splint	Compression Sleeves
2		Strassburg Sock	
1 – Least Effective	Topical Pain Reduction Creams (Voltaren)		Losing Weight

Treatment Categories

There are numerous treatment options for plantar fasciitis. They are divided into different categories based on the purpose of the treatment. There are 3 purposes of treatment.

1. **Reducing Inflammation** - These treatments focus on reducing the inflammation that is the main reason for the pain you are feeling. If you do not reduce the inflammation, you may continue to limp and walk differently, which can cause pain to other parts of your foot or your body.

2. **Reducing Tightness** - This is focusing on reducing tightness of the fascia on the bottom of the foot, and more importantly, reducing tightness to the muscles that are on the back of your leg that insert either into the heel region or the foot. Tightness is the most misunderstood reason for plantar fasciitis.

3. **Stabilizing Foot & Reducing Pressure** - Stabilizing the foot is essential for your foot to work better. If you have a foot that is flat or pronated, it becomes unstable. As a result, the muscles in the foot and the back of the leg region must work harder. The more stable your foot becomes the less work you must put into walking and being active. Reducing pressure is the least important aspect of treatment, in my opinion. If you have plantar fasciitis in only one foot and they both have the same pressure on them, why don't they both hurt the same? Reducing the pressure can help initially but only if there is inflammation (as mentioned in item number one), but once the inflammation is improved, there is less of a need to reduce pressure on the heel region.

After each treatment you will find an explanation of the treatment as well as the "Pros" and "Cons" of each to help you better decide what is the best for you.

Reduce Inflammation

- Cortisone Injection: Many times, a corticosteroid injection can help reduce the inflammation and pain around the plantar fascia.

  Pros: For some patients this can resolve the issue of plantar fasciitis very quickly and minimize additional treatment.

  Cons: Usually you can only have 3 injections per location per year. These injections can weaken the fascia, and delay the use of other treatments because of the effects on inflammation.

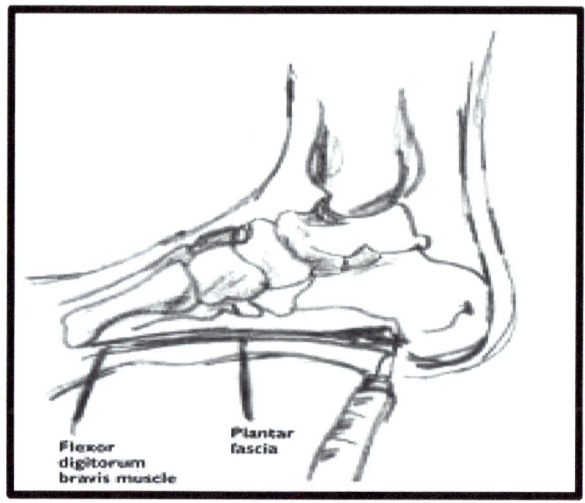

Figure 4:Example of placement of cortisone injection

- Shockwave therapy (EPAT): This is a non-invasive surgical procedure that uses high intensity sound waves to break up adhesions on the plantar fascia and to help activate your body's healing response.

  Pros: You can avoid having a cortisone injection and may resolve the heel pain. There are no side effects with the treatments, and there is less need for time off work following the procedure.

Cons: Sometimes it is not powerful enough to reduce inflammation and can be painful for some patients. Usually it is not a covered procedure under most insurance plans.

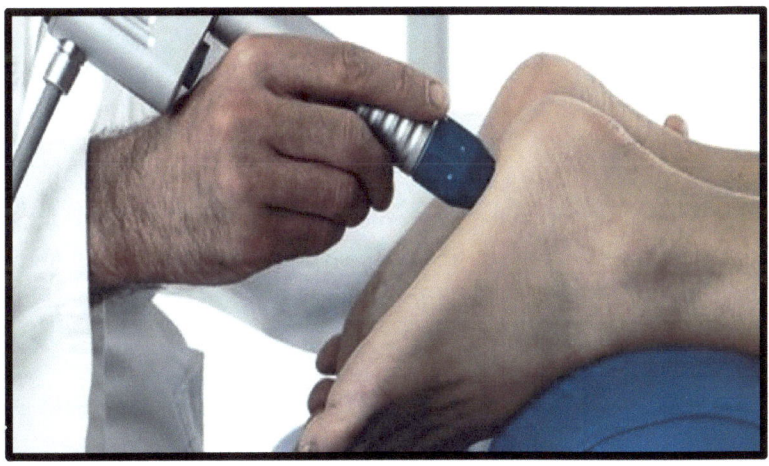

Figure 5: Example of shockwave treatment for plantar fasciitis

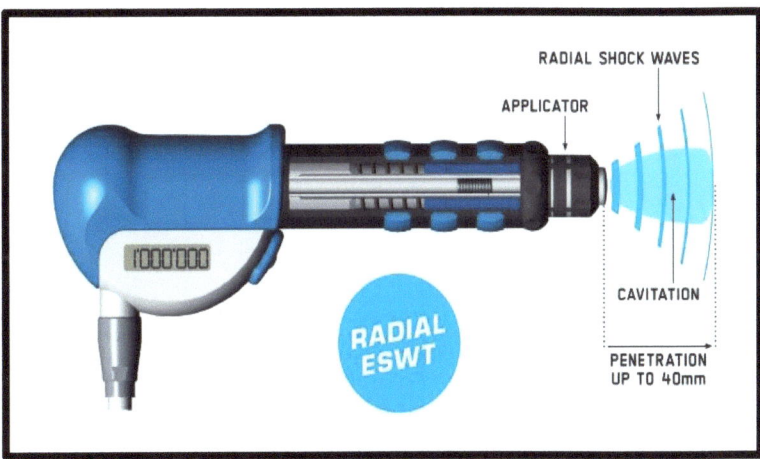

Figure 6: Example of shockwave handpeice

- <u>Amniotic Membrane Therapy:</u> This is an injection that is done under ultrasound guidance into the area of maximal pain and inflammation. This therapy uses amniotic cells to help regulate inflammation in the body.

  <u>Pros:</u> This is a good alternative to surgery and can greatly reduce inflammation naturally.

  <u>Cons:</u> Usually is not a covered treatment under most insurance plans.

- <u>Medications:</u> Oral anti-inflammatory drugs (NSAIDs), such as Ibuprofen, may help reduce pain and inflammation. Also, there are steroid-type medications such as Prednisone that can help reduce inflammation.

  <u>Pros:</u> These can help reduce inflammation for low level pain and inflammation.

  <u>Cons:</u> Some people cannot take them due to stomach issues and they can cause other health conditions if taken long term. Also, they are not as effective as a cortisone injection.

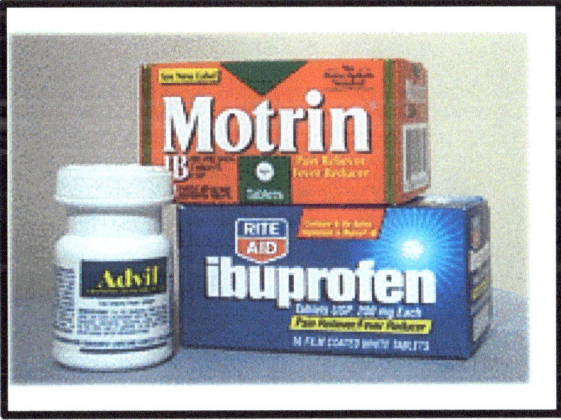

Figure 7: Example of different anti-inflammatory medications

- Ice: Putting an ice pack on your heel for 10 minutes a few times a day helps reduce the inflammation. An easy method of icing is using a frozen bottle of water to massage the bottom of your foot.

Pros: This is easy to do on the foot and heel region.

Cons: Many people find it less effective than a cortisone injection, and it tends to make the area feel better only while icing. It is less helpful for more longstanding plantar fasciitis or more severe symptoms.

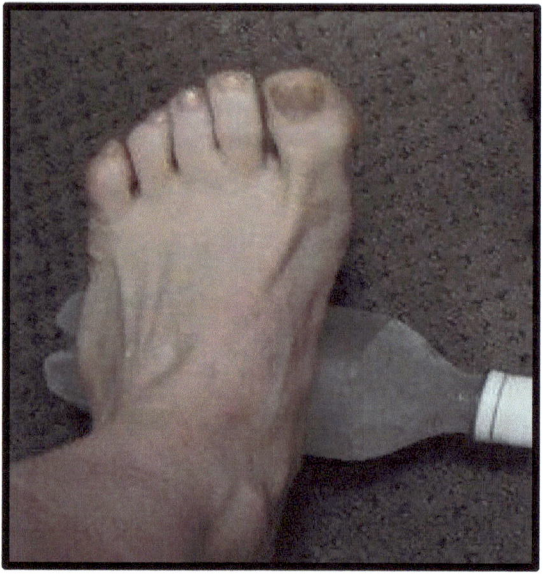

Figure 8: How to ice the bottom of the foot with water bottle

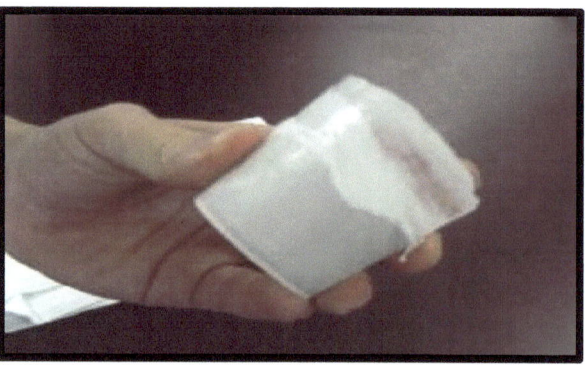

Figure 9: Method of icing with a paper cup

- <u>Contrast Bath:</u> Another way to reduce inflammation is to switch from a bucket of cold water to hot water as this can help reduce the inflammation. Switch from one basin to another every 5 minutes ending on the cold.

<u>Pros:</u> This can help reset the pain signals in your foot and ankle by causing vasoconstriction and vasodilation in the foot area, thus reducing swelling and pain.

<u>Cons:</u> It is time consuming.

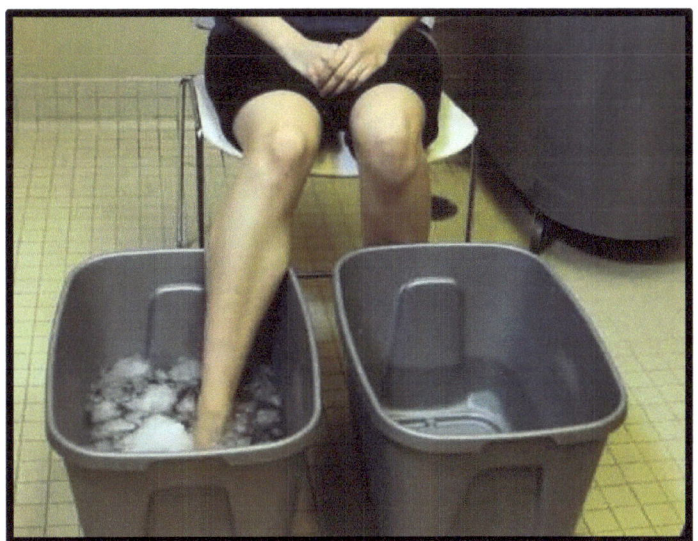

Figure 10: Contrast bath example

- <u>Platelet Rich Plasma:</u> The plasma portion of our natural blood has many healing components. This procedure uses the patient's own blood in a concentrated form and injects it into the area of injury on the plantar fascia. Following the procedure, the patient is immobilized in a removable walking cast and needs minimal time off work.

<u>Pros:</u> Uses your own blood platelets to reduce inflammation.

<u>Cons:</u> Expensive and conflicting research about the treatment.

- <u>Topical Pain Creams</u>: There are many compounded creams that are available to help with reducing pain and inflammation. Some are purchased over the counter and others are prescribed.

  <u>Pros:</u> They cannot be taken by mouth or injection.

  <u>Cons:</u> These topical treatments are usually the least effective if you have much pain with your plantar fasciitis.

Reduce Tightness

- <u>Physical therapy:</u> When stretching alone is not enough, either home physical therapy tools or a physical therapy evaluation may be beneficial.

  <u>Pros:</u> Most patients who have physical therapy get better quicker and people are more consistent at doing home exercises with a therapist due to accountability.

  <u>Cons:</u> There are some people who don't get better with physical therapy and it can be expensive if you have a high-deductible healthcare plan.

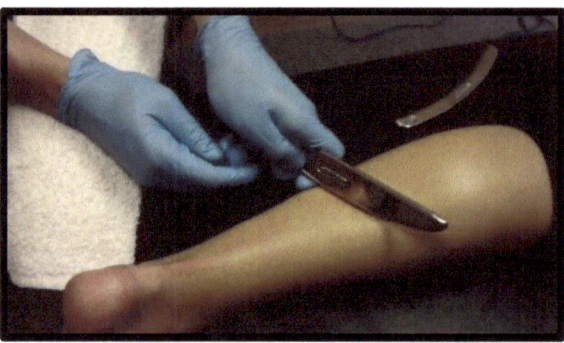

Figure 11: Example of graston technique modality for physical therapy

- Trigger Point: Deep tissue massage using trigger point tools is a dynamic treatment option as compared to static stretching exercises. The basis is on reducing soft tissue adhesions to the muscles in the back of the leg that can lead to heel pain. This treatment can be done in the convenience of your home with quick results. These can include a trigger point ball, foam roller or stick roller.

Pros: Effective if used at home and if used properly. Works better if you track your home therapy.

Cons: You need to be motivated to use the trigger point tools and make sure you learn to use them correctly. Still, not as good as physical therapy in terms of effectiveness.

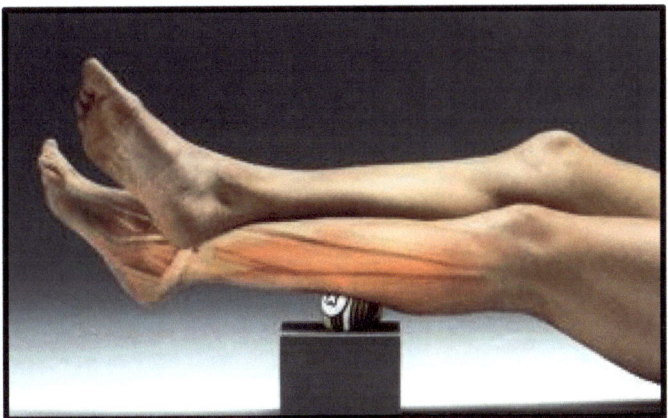

Figure 12: Example of block with roller ball for back of calf region

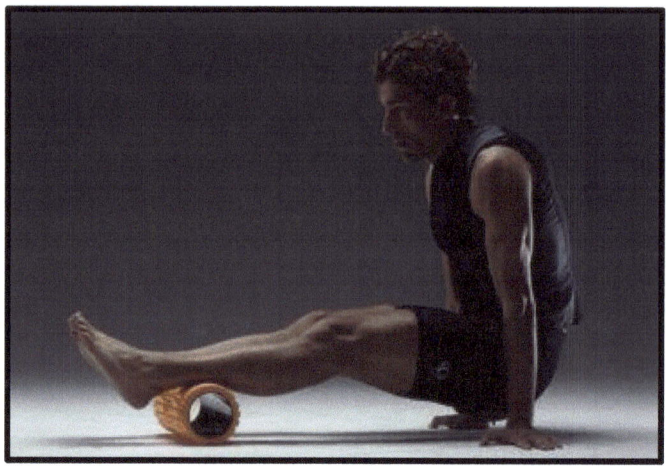

Figure 13: Example of foam rolling back of calf region

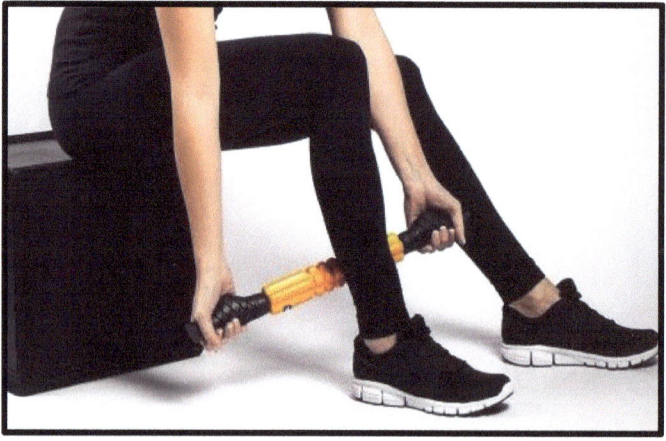

Figure 14: Example of using "stick" roller for back of calf region

- <u>Stretching exercises:</u> Exercises that stretch out the calf muscles and the plantar fascia can help ease the pain and assist with recovery. However, I prefer the deep tissue massage tools over stretching that are discussed later in this book.

Pros: Easy to do anywhere you are without any tools.

Cons: Many people stretch incorrectly and can overstretch causing more problems. Less effective than physical therapy or other tools that are used.

- Night splint: Wearing a night splint allows you to passively stretch your plantar fascia and calf muscles while sleeping. This can help reduce the morning pain experienced by some patients. This is an effective treatment when used with non-custom orthotics to prevent foot flattening (pronation) while in the night splint.

Pros: This is very helpful if you have morning pain with the first step out of bed in the morning.

Cons: If you are a belly sleeper this may not work for you. Also, for some patients they cannot tolerate it the whole night and end up removing it in the middle of the night. Another way to use the brace is at the end of your day while watching TV at night. There is another type of splint called an Anterior Night Splint that goes on the front of the foot that may work better in that case.

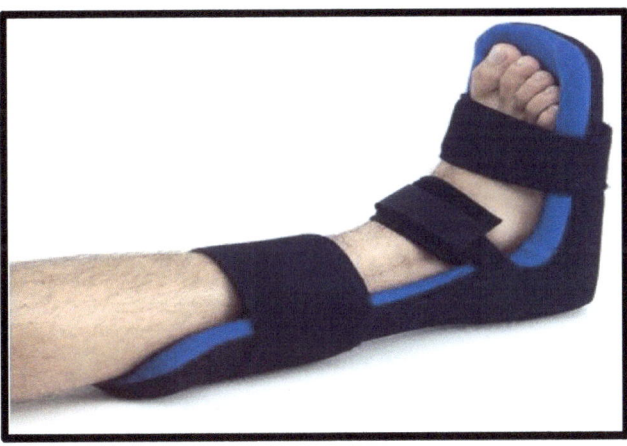

Figure 15: Example of night splint

- Strassburg Sock: this type of a treatment is like a night splint but holds your foot while flexed in the upward direction while sleeping. For some people this is more comfortable than a night splint.

Pros: Like the night splint, this can help with pain with the first step getting up in the morning.

Cons: Can cause toe numbness for some patients due to the amount of pulling up on the toes. Also, this pulls on the toes and does not do as good of a job at dorsiflexing the whole foot.

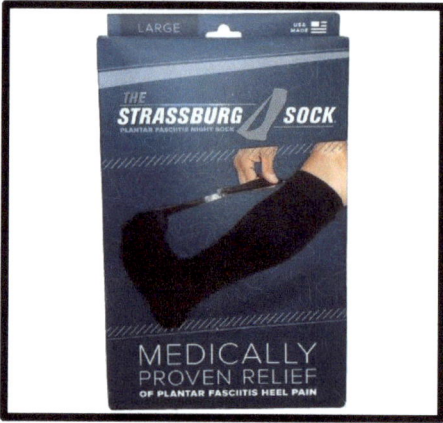

Figure 16: Example of Strassburg Sock

Stabilizing Foot & Reduce Pressure

- Custom Orthotic Devices: Custom orthotic devices are specially molded to your foot and help correct the underlying structural abnormalities causing the plantar fasciitis. These are used to support the arch region but more importantly, they are used to correct the heel alignment. As you can see with the picture below, the heel position is more aligned after the orthotics are placed on the patient. The big difference between inserts you purchase at the store is that they do not correct the heel position as well as a custom-made device. However, a custom orthotic can be 5-10 times more expensive than an over-the-counter device.

<u>Pros:</u> If made correctly for your condition, it can help reduce pain and prevent recurrence of the condition. Custom orthotics usually last 5-10 years, much longer than shoes or inserts.

<u>Cons:</u> If this is not fit or made to your foot, you may not be able to wear the device. Many times, custom orthotics take weeks to break in and feel comfortable. You may need to wear a less supportive shoe due to all the support in the orthotic. Many times, custom orthotics are not covered by insurance and can cost between $300-600.

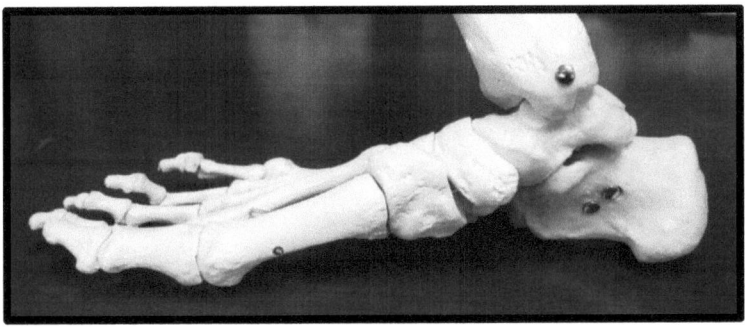

Figure 17: Example of pronated foot or foot with lower arch

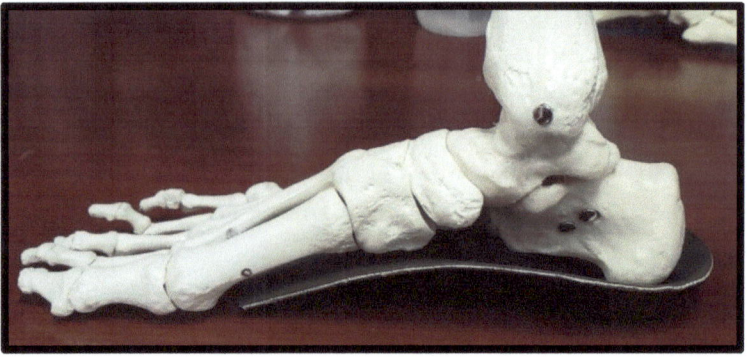

Figure 18: Example of foot with arch corrected by orthotic

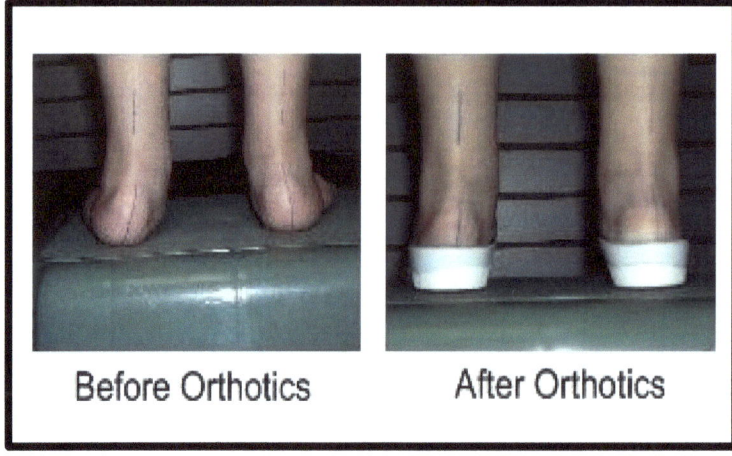

Figure 19: Example of corrected heel position with orthotics

- <u>Removable Walking Boot:</u> In more severe cases wearing a walking cast boot for a few weeks can allow your foot to rest and heal. This boot can help your foot, muscles, and tendons on the back of the calf region rest.

  <u>Pros:</u> This boot is easy to wear and can make you slow down if you are very active. It is not made to wear for a long period of time but for many people can help with pain.

Cons: You cannot drive with this boot if your right foot is injured. The boot has a little lift to it and sometimes you need another device called an Even-Up. The Even-Up is worn on the non-injured foot, over your shoe, to bring you to the same height as the boot. Or you may prefer to wear a shoe with a heel so that you do not develop knee, hip or back pain while wearing the walking boot.

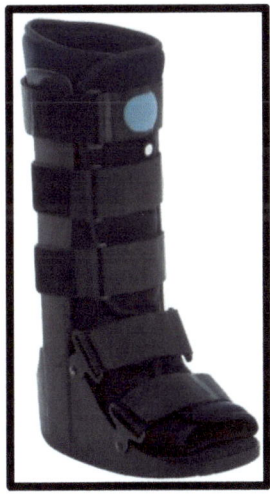

Figure 20: Walking boot

- Arch supports: Over-the-counter arch supports are non-specific to your foot type. They may help some people and are a good place to start treating heel pain. Keep in mind that unless you have new supportive shoes, arch supports will not help.

  Pros: Less expensive than custom orthotics and for many people they can give enough support to help with heel pain.

  Cons: Very rigid and some people with a very inflamed foot can find them uncomfortable. They are not custom orthotics, so if you have much pronation or your heel is tilted, they will not correct the foot as much as a custom orthotic.

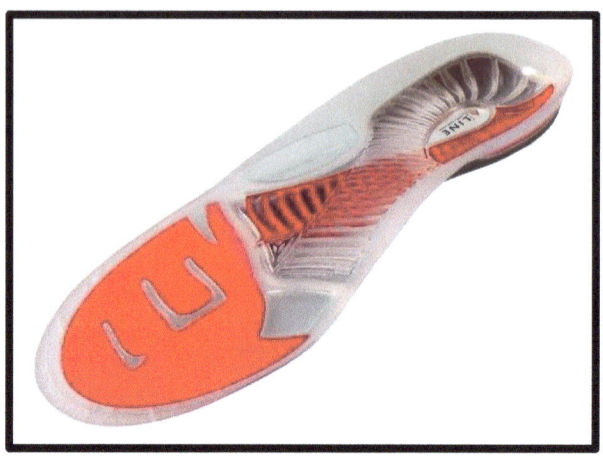

Figure 21: Rigid orthotic example

- <u>Shoes</u>: Wearing supportive shoes that have good arch support and a slightly raised heel can help reduce the stress on the plantar fascia. When buying shoes, they should be comfortable from the moment you buy them. Make sure you shop for shoes at the end of your day when your feet are the largest. A good shoe that is popular now is a Hoka shoe that has extra cushion to the bottom of the foot. There are many shoes that are marketed to be for "plantar fasciitis", but this is only marketing. If you have quite a bit of pain and no shoe is comfortable, buying another one will probably not help. You should focus more on reducing inflammation with other treatments as explained elsewhere in this book.

<u>Pros:</u> Hoka shoes are very supportive and have great stability and cushioning. Many people find them comfortable.

<u>Cons:</u> Hoka shoes are elevated from the ground as a platform shoe

and some people who wear these shoes have balance issues.

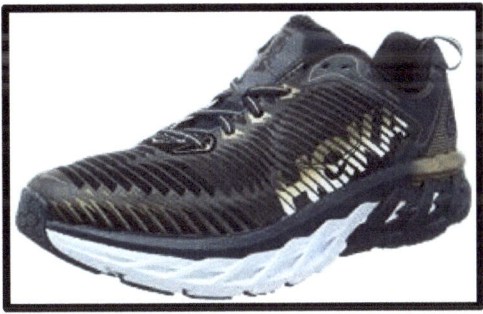

Figure 22: Hoka shoe example

- <u>Supportive flip-flops</u>: It is best to have a flip-flop that has good support in the arch region. Also, try to avoid going barefoot. When you walk without shoes you put undue strain and stress on the plantar fascia.

  <u>Pros:</u> These offer more support to the arch region than a traditional flip-flop.
  <u>Cons:</u> The flip-flops that are more supportive usually don't look as good as other ones.

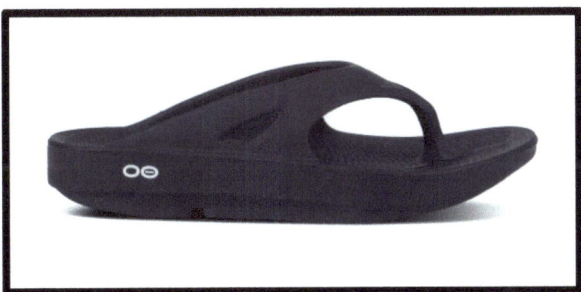

Figure 23: Oofos sandal

- Strapping: Consists of placing padding and tape on the bottom of the foot to help support the foot and reduce the strain on the plantar fascia. Here is an example of the tape that will work well for strapping your foot.

  Pros: This can help support your foot and reduce pain by increasing support.
  Cons: This is cumbersome to do on your own and makes it difficult to shower.

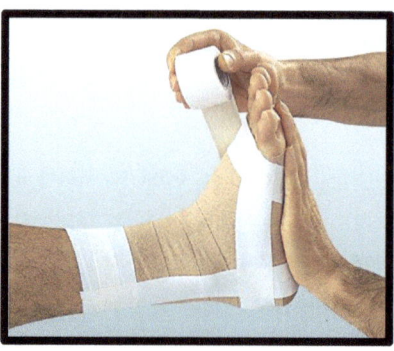

Figure 24: Strapping or foot taping example

- Padding: An Aircast Airheel pad can be placed under the heel to help minimize the pain. However, correction of the mechanical abnormality is still necessary. I don't recommend simply using an insert made of gel or just a cushion. It may make you feel better in the short-term but does not provide any correction of your foot and will not help long-term.

  Pros: This works well if you have lots of heel pain but there are other treatments that work better to reduce the inflammation.

  Cons: This usually is not worn long-term and there are other treatments that are more beneficial.

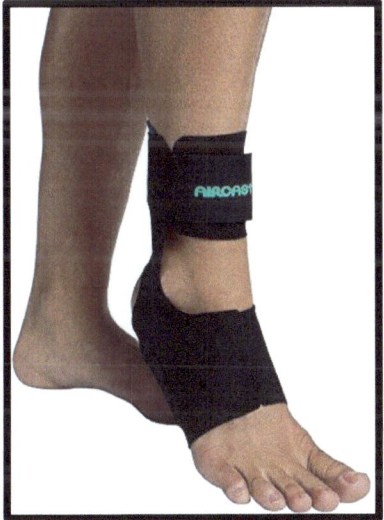

Figure 25: Aircast Airheel

- <u>Compression Sleeve</u>: Many patients with plantar fasciitis feel better with additional compression on the foot. This is similar, but not the same, as taping the foot. There are compression sleeves that work very well for this.

  <u>Pros:</u> Compression sleeves can offer support similarly to strapping, as noted before, and they can be removed and placed on again.

  <u>Cons:</u> They can be a little expensive or bothersome because they are very tight.

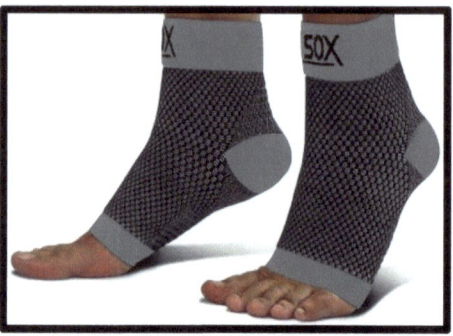

Figure 26: Compression Sleeve (Socks)

- Lose weight: Reducing extra pounds will help decrease the strain on the plantar fascia. Many people come into the office with plantar fasciitis because they are exercising to lose weight. There is a new concept I am sharing with many of my patients called "Intermittent Fasting."

  Pros: This can help in general and will reduce pressure on your feet, but weight loss by itself rarely cures plantar fasciitis.

  Cons: **None!**

Surgical Options

Although **most patients with plantar fasciitis respond well to non-surgical treatments,** a small percentage of patients may require more advanced or surgical treatments. If, after many months of conservative treatment, you continue to have pain, these are other options that can be considered:

- Endoscopic plantar fasciotomy: This is a procedure that uses a small incision to identify and then surgically cut a portion of the plantar fascia to help relieve the pain.

Pros: Smaller incision and quicker recovery.

Cons: Sometimes results in nerve injury and   sometimes does not resolve the problem of the plantar fascial pain.

- Open plantar fasciotomy: this procedure is like the one above except that a larger incision is made.

Pros: Easier to see the fascia and cut through a portion of the fascia.

Cons: Larger incision usually a little longer recovery. Sometimes does not resolve the problem of the plantar fascial pain.

Preventing Plantar Fasciitis

No matter what type of treatment is used to treat plantar fasciitis, the **underlying causes that led to this condition may remain.** Therefore, you will need to continue with preventative measures such as soft tissue work to the back of the calf region, supportive shoes and custom orthotic devices for long-term treatment of plantar fasciitis.   Recurrence is common, especially when using cortisone injections if no other treatment is done. The cortisone injection can reduce the inflammation temporarily, but if no other treatment is used, the inflammation can quickly return.

Plantar Fasciitis Treatment Checklist

Here is a checklist you can use with your doctor to go over the different treatment options for treating your plantar fasciitis.

The Plantar Fasciitis Checklist

Imaging

- ❏ X-ray
- ❏ Diagnostic Ultrasound
- ❏ MRI

Traditional Treatments

Reduce Inflammation

- ❏ Cortisone Injection (8 weeks)
- ❏ Shockwave Therapy (EPAT)
- ❏ Amnio Injection
- ❏ NSAIDs and Prednisone
- ❏ Icing & Contrast Baths

Reduce Tightness

- ❏ Physical Therapy

- ❏ Home Therapy - Foam Rolling
- ❏ Stretching
- ❏ Night Splint

Stabilize Foot - Reduce Pressure

- ❏ Custom Orthotics
- ❏ Walking Boot
- ❏ Arch Support
- ❏ Supportive Shoes
- ❏ Heel Cup

Over 12 Months

Surgery

Second Opinion

Figure 27: The plantar fasciitis checklist

Frequently Asked Questions

Q: Do I need orthotics to get rid of plantar fasciitis?

A: Each patient is different. Even though the pain may subside, the mechanical instability and excess movement of the foot that caused the problem still needs to be addressed. Using supportive shoes and orthotics are very effective at controlling foot motion.

Q: Will I need surgery for plantar fasciitis?

A: Most of our patients DO NOT advance to surgery due to plantar fasciitis. However, if you have been treated for six months to a year with no improvement, then some surgical options may be considered.

Q: When should I seek treatment for plantar fasciitis?

A: Since there are so many home treatment options to try, that is a good place to start. However, keep in mind that seeing a doctor can help you get better faster than on your own. If you have had it for over a month and it is not improving with the home treatments, it is best to make an appointment.

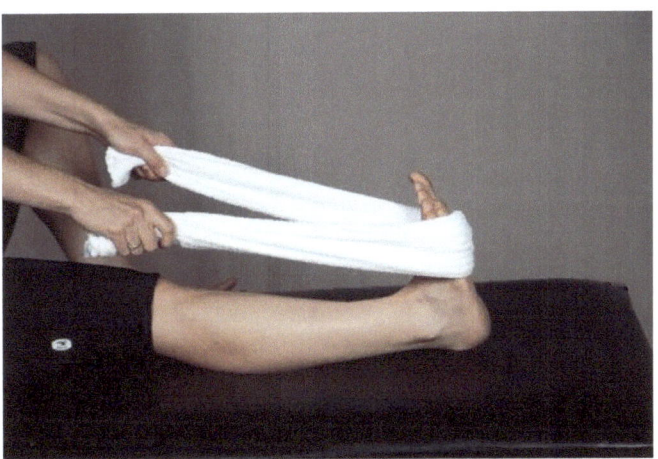

Figure 28: Towel stretching for morning pain reduction

Q: How do I reduce the pain I have in the morning when getting up?

A: The best way to reduce the pain in the morning when getting up is to either sleep with a night splint on your leg or stretch with a towel for a few minutes before getting up out of bed. Finally, you can put on a shoe or a sandal first thing out of bed to reduce the pain when getting out of bed.

Additional Resources

If you have found this helpful and would like to learn more about plantar fasciitis, I have put together a course of plantar fasciitis that can be very helpful. There are many more downloads and way of tracking your progress.

To view about other learning resources about plantar fasciitis, go to www.drpelto.thinkific.com.

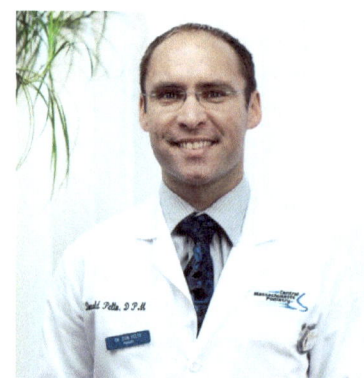

Conclusion

I hope you have enjoyed these resources for treating your plantar fasciitis. My desire with this book is to provide the best usable information for treating your plantar fasciitis. These resources can be used on your own for self-treatment or if you are seeing a specialist.

To your health,

Dr. Donald Pelto

www.ingramcontent.com/pod-product-compliance
Lightning Source LLC
Chambersburg PA
CBHW041210180526
45172CB00006B/1226